ZYN KNIGHT HARRIS

Fuck like a pornstar : The male guide to sexual health

This book was professionally typeset on Reedsy.
Find out more at reedsy.com

"Dedicated to all individuals who believe in the power of knowledge, communication, and empowerment in achieving and maintaining optimal sexual health and well-being. May this book serve as a valuable guide, offering insights, resources, and support on the journey toward a fulfilling and satisfying sexual life. Here's to embracing sexual wellness, fostering healthy relationships, and advocating for inclusive, equitable sexual healthcare for all."

"Sexual health is an essential component of overall well-being, deserving of understanding, attention, and proactive care. Let's embark on a journey of knowledge, empowerment, and advocacy to nurture fulfilling and satisfying sexual lives for ourselves and others."

Contents

Foreword

Welcome to a comprehensive guide dedicated to exploring the intricate facets of sexual health and well-being. In today's world, where conversations about sexual health can often be shrouded in stigma or misinformation, this book stands as a beacon of clarity, knowledge, and empowerment.

Sexual health encompasses not just physical aspects but also emotional, mental, and relational dimensions. It is about understanding our bodies, embracing our desires, fostering healthy communication, and seeking support when needed. Through this book, readers will embark on a journey of self-discovery, education, and empowerment in navigating the complexities of sexual wellness.

As society continues to evolve, so too do our perspectives on sexuality, relationships, and personal fulfillment. This book embraces diversity, inclusivity, and the recognition that every individual's journey toward sexual health is unique. It provides a wealth of information, resources, and practical advice to help readers make informed choices, address challenges, and cultivate positive sexual experiences.

The chapters within this book cover a wide array of topics, from understanding the fundamentals of sexual health to exploring techniques for enhancing pleasure, managing challenges, and accessing support. Each chapter is crafted to provide valuable insights, actionable strategies, and a compassionate approach to sexual well-being.

I encourage readers to approach this book with an open mind, a willingness to learn, and a commitment to prioritizing their sexual health and that of their partners. Remember, sexual health is a vital aspect of overall well-being, and by embracing knowledge, communication, and self-care, we can all strive to lead healthier, happier lives.

May this book serve as a trusted companion on your journey toward sexual wellness and fulfillment.

Warm regards,

Zyn Knight Harris

Preface

Welcome to "Fuck like a pornstar : The male guide to sexual health" This book is a culmination of extensive research, expert insights, and a deep commitment to promoting holistic sexual well-being for individuals of all backgrounds and experiences.

Sexual health is an integral part of human life, encompassing physical, emotional, mental, and social aspects. However, discussions surrounding sexual health often carry stigma, confusion, or lack of accurate information. This book aims to bridge those gaps by providing reliable, accessible, and empowering guidance on navigating the complexities of sexual wellness.

As the author of this book, I have drawn upon the expertise of healthcare professionals, sexual health advocates, and individuals with lived experiences to create a comprehensive resource that addresses a wide range of topics. From understanding the basics of sexual anatomy and function to exploring strategies for enhancing pleasure, managing challenges, and accessing support services, each chapter is designed to inform, educate, and empower readers.

Throughout these pages, you will find evidence-based information, practical tips, self-assessment tools, and resources to support your journey toward optimal sexual health. Whether you are seeking guidance on contraception, STI prevention, communication skills, or sexual pleasure techniques, this book is crafted to meet your needs with compassion, exclusivity, and respect for individual diversity.

It is my sincere hope that this book serves as a trusted companion on your path to sexual wellness and empowerment. By embracing knowledge, open communication, self-care, and advocacy, we can create a world where everyone has the resources and support they need to lead fulfilling, satisfying, and healthy sexual lives.

I invite you to embark on this journey with curiosity, an open heart, and a commitment to prioritizing your sexual health and well-being. Together, let us explore, learn, and empower ourselves to embrace the fullness of our sexual selves.

Warm regards,

Zyn Knight Harris

Acknowledgement

Writing a book on such a nuanced and essential topic as sexual health requires the collaboration, support, and expertise of many individuals and organizations. I extend my heartfelt gratitude to everyone who has contributed to the creation of this comprehensive guide to sexual wellness and empowerment.

First and foremost, I am immensely grateful to the healthcare professionals, sexual health experts, and researchers whose knowledge and insights have informed the content of this book. Your dedication to advancing sexual health education and advocacy is truly admirable, and I am honored to incorporate your expertise into these pages.

I would also like to thank the individuals who shared their personal experiences, stories, and perspectives on sexual health. Your courage, openness, and willingness to contribute to this project have added depth, authenticity, and relatability to the discussions within this book.

A special acknowledgment goes to the advocacy organizations, community centers, and support groups that tirelessly work to promote sexual health, destigmatize sexual topics, and provide invaluable resources to individuals seeking information and support. Your commitment to inclusivity, accessibility, and empowerment is reflected in the resources and recommendations included in this book.

I extend my appreciation to the publishers, editors, designers, and everyone involved in the production process of this book. Your dedication to ensuring the accuracy, clarity, and professionalism of the content has been instrumental in bringing this project to fruition.

Lastly, I express my gratitude to the readers of this book. Your curiosity, engagement, and commitment to prioritizing sexual health and well-being inspire me to continue advocating for comprehensive sexual education, open communication, and empowerment for all.

Thank you to each and every individual and organization that has contributed to this book. Your contributions have made a difference in promoting positive attitudes, knowledge, and access to sexual health resources, and I am deeply grateful for your support.

Warm regards,

Zyn Knight Harris

Chapter 1: Understanding Male Sexual Health

In this chapter, we will delve into the intricate mechanisms of male sexual health, exploring the anatomy involved, the stages of the sexual response cycle, common sexual health issues, and their underlying causes.

Male Anatomy and Physiology

The male reproductive system is a complex network of organs and hormones that work together to facilitate sexual function and reproduction. Central to this system are the penis, testes, prostate gland, and a series of ducts and glands that produce and transport sperm and semen.

1. **Penis**: The penis is the primary external sexual organ in males. It consists of three cylindrical bodies of spongy tissue, known as the corpora cavernosa and corpus spongiosum, which become engorged with blood during sexual arousal, leading to an erection.
2. **Testes**: The testes, or testicles, are responsible for producing sperm and testosterone, the primary male sex hormone. Sperm production

occurs within the seminiferous tubules of the testes, while testosterone is synthesized by Leydig cells.

3. **Prostate Gland**: The prostate gland is a small, walnut-sized gland located below the bladder. It produces seminal fluid, a milky substance that nourishes and transports sperm during ejaculation.
4. **Seminal Vesicles and Ejaculatory Ducts**: These structures contribute additional fluids to semen and play a role in the ejaculation process.

The Sexual Response Cycle

Understanding the sexual response cycle is essential for comprehending male sexual function and dysfunction. The cycle consists of four phases:

1. **Excitement Phase**: This phase is characterized by sexual arousal, initiated by physical or psychological stimuli. Blood flow to the genitals increases, leading to erection and lubrication.
2. **Plateau Phase**: During this phase, arousal continues to intensify, and muscle tension builds throughout the body. The penis becomes fully erect, and the testicles may elevate closer to the body.
3. **Orgasmic Phase**: The orgasmic phase is marked by intense pleasure and rhythmic contractions of the pelvic muscles. Ejaculation typically occurs during this phase, accompanied by the release of semen.
4. **Resolution Phase**: After orgasm, the body gradually returns to its pre-aroused state. Erection subsides, and heart rate, blood pressure, and breathing return to normal levels.

Common Sexual Health Issues

Several factors can impact male sexual health, leading to various issues that may affect sexual function and satisfaction. Some of the common sexual health issues include:

1. **Erectile Dysfunction (ED)**: ED refers to the inability to achieve or

maintain an erection sufficient for sexual activity. It can result from physical causes such as vascular problems, hormonal imbalances, or psychological factors like stress and anxiety.

2. **Premature Ejaculation (PE)**: PE is characterized by ejaculating sooner than desired, often leading to distress or relationship difficulties. Psychological factors, hypersensitivity, or abnormal reflex activity may contribute to PE.

3. **Low Libido (Hypoactive Sexual Desire Disorder)**: Decreased sexual desire or interest can stem from hormonal imbalances, relationship issues, stress, depression, or certain medications.

4. **Delayed Ejaculation**: This condition involves difficulty or delay in reaching orgasm and ejaculating, which can be linked to psychological factors, medication side effects, or neurological issues.

5. **Prostate Problems**: Conditions such as prostatitis or benign prostatic hyperplasia (BPH) can affect urinary and sexual function in men, leading to symptoms like pain, discomfort, and erectile difficulties.

Understanding the Causes

To effectively address sexual health issues, it's crucial to identify and understand their underlying causes. These causes can be categorized as physical, psychological, or a combination of both:

1. **Physical Causes**:

- **Vascular Issues**: Conditions that affect blood flow, such as cardiovascular disease, diabetes, or hypertension, can contribute to erectile dysfunction.
- **Hormonal Imbalances**: Reduced testosterone levels or imbalances in other hormones can impact libido and sexual function.
- **Neurological Conditions**: Disorders affecting the nervous system, such as multiple sclerosis or spinal cord injuries, may interfere with sexual response.

- **Medication Side Effects**: Some medications, including antidepressants, antihypertensives, and prostate medications, can affect sexual function as a side effect.
- **Chronic Illnesses**: Conditions like kidney disease, liver cirrhosis, or chronic obstructive pulmonary disease (COPD) can impact overall health, including sexual function.

1. **Psychological Causes**:

- **Stress and Anxiety**: High levels of stress, anxiety, or performance pressure can hinder sexual arousal and function.
- **Depression**: Mood disorders like depression can reduce libido and lead to sexual difficulties.
- **Relationship Issues**: Conflicts, communication problems, or lack of intimacy within relationships can affect sexual desire and satisfaction.
- **Past Trauma or Abuse**: Previous traumatic experiences or abuse can have long-lasting effects on sexual health and functioning.

1. **Lifestyle Factors**:

- **Smoking**: Tobacco use can damage blood vessels and impair circulation, contributing to erectile problems.
- **Alcohol and Drug Use**: Excessive alcohol consumption or drug use can interfere with sexual performance and libido.
- **Poor Diet and Exercise**: Unhealthy eating habits and sedentary lifestyle can impact overall health, including sexual function.
- **Sleep Disorders**: Lack of quality sleep or sleep disorders like sleep apnea can affect hormonal balance and sexual health.

Conclusion

Understanding male sexual health involves a comprehensive exploration of anatomy, physiology, the sexual response cycle, common issues, and their underlying causes. By gaining insight into these aspects, individuals can take proactive steps to maintain or improve their sexual well-being, seek appropriate medical care when needed, and enhance their overall quality of life.

Two

Chapter 2: Mental and Emotional Health

In this chapter, we will explore the intricate connection between mental and emotional health and male sexual well-being. We'll delve into the impact of stress, anxiety, depression, and other psychological factors on libido, sexual performance, and overall sexual satisfaction. Additionally, we'll discuss strategies and techniques for managing mental and emotional health to improve sexual function and quality of life.

The Mind-Body Connection

The relationship between mental and emotional health and sexual function is profound and multifaceted. Psychological factors can significantly influence sexual desire, arousal, performance, and overall sexual satisfaction. Understanding this mind-body connection is crucial for addressing sexual health issues effectively.

1. **Stress and Anxiety**:

- **Impact on Libido**: High levels of stress and anxiety can diminish libido and sexual desire. The body's stress response, characterized by increased cortisol levels, can interfere with hormonal balance and sexual arousal.

- **Performance Anxiety**: Fear of performance failure or concerns about sexual performance can lead to anxiety during sexual encounters, contributing to erectile difficulties or premature ejaculation.
- **Coping Mechanisms**: Developing healthy coping mechanisms for stress and anxiety, such as mindfulness techniques, relaxation exercises, or therapy, can positively impact sexual well-being.

1. **Depression and Mood Disorders**:

- **Libido and Interest**: Depression can decrease libido and interest in sexual activities. Symptoms such as fatigue, low self-esteem, and loss of pleasure (anhedonia) can also affect sexual function.
- **Medication Side Effects**: Some antidepressant medications may have sexual side effects, including decreased libido, erectile dysfunction, or delayed ejaculation. Consulting a healthcare provider about medication options is essential.
- **Holistic Treatment**: Treating depression and mood disorders holistically, through therapy, medication management, lifestyle changes, and social support, can improve overall well-being, including sexual health.

Coping Strategies and Techniques

1. **Mindfulness and Relaxation**:

- **Mindfulness Practices**: Mindfulness meditation, deep breathing exercises, and progressive muscle relaxation techniques can help reduce stress, anxiety, and promote a sense of calmness and presence during sexual activities.
- **Yoga and Tai Chi**: Incorporating mind-body practices like yoga or tai chi into daily routines can enhance relaxation, flexibility, and overall well-being, contributing to better sexual health.

1. **Communication and Connection**:

- **Open Communication**: Discussing sexual concerns, desires, and preferences with partners in a non-judgmental and supportive manner can strengthen intimacy and enhance sexual satisfaction.
- **Emotional Connection**: Building emotional intimacy through meaningful conversations, shared experiences, and acts of affection can deepen the bond between partners and improve sexual experiences.

1. **Healthy Lifestyle Choices**:

- **Regular Exercise**: Engaging in regular physical activity not only improves cardiovascular health and stamina but also boosts mood, reduces stress, and enhances self-confidence, all of which contribute to better sexual function.
- **Balanced Diet**: Consuming a balanced diet rich in fruits, vegetables, lean proteins, and whole grains provides essential nutrients for overall health, including sexual health. Limiting processed foods, sugar, and alcohol can also benefit sexual function.
- **Adequate Sleep**: Prioritizing quality sleep and establishing healthy sleep habits can regulate hormone levels, improve mood, and increase energy levels, all of which are vital for sexual well-being.

1. **Stress Management**:

- **Stress Reduction Techniques**: Engage in activities that promote relaxation and stress reduction, such as hobbies, spending time in nature, listening to music, or practicing mindfulness.
- **Time Management**: Effective time management strategies can reduce feelings of overwhelm and create space for self-care, relaxation, and leisure activities, which are essential for mental and emotional well-being.

Seeking Professional Support

Sometimes, managing mental and emotional health concerns may require professional support and intervention. It's essential to recognize when to seek help from mental health professionals, such as therapists, counselors, or psychiatrists, especially if symptoms significantly impact daily functioning, relationships, or quality of life.

1. **Therapy and Counseling**:

- **Individual Therapy**: Cognitive-behavioral therapy (CBT), mindfulness-based therapies, and psychodynamic approaches can help address underlying psychological factors contributing to sexual health issues.
- **Couples Counseling**: Relationship-focused therapy can improve communication, intimacy, and sexual satisfaction within partnerships.

1. **Medication Management**:

- **Antidepressants and Mood Stabilizers**: In cases where medication is necessary for managing depression, anxiety, or other mood disorders, working closely with a healthcare provider to monitor and adjust medication can minimize sexual side effects.

1. **Support Groups**:

- **Peer Support**: Participating in support groups or online forums focused on mental health, sexuality, or specific concerns can provide validation, insights, and a sense of community during challenging times.

Conclusion

Mental and emotional health profoundly influence male sexual well-being, affecting libido, arousal, performance, and overall sexual satisfaction. By recognizing the interconnectedness of mind and body, implementing coping strategies, fostering healthy lifestyle habits, and seeking appropriate professional support when needed, individuals can enhance their mental, emotional, and sexual health, leading to a more fulfilling and satisfying life.

Three

Chapter 3: Nutrition and Diet

This chapter explores the vital role of nutrition and diet in male sexual health. We will delve into the impact of dietary choices on libido, erectile function, hormonal balance, and overall sexual well-being. Understanding how nutrition influences physiological processes related to sexual health can empower individuals to make informed dietary decisions that support optimal sexual function.

Nutrients Essential for Sexual Health

1. **Macronutrients**:

- **Proteins**: Protein-rich foods such as lean meats, poultry, fish, legumes, and tofu provide essential amino acids necessary for hormone production, muscle function, and overall vitality.
- **Carbohydrates**: Complex carbohydrates from whole grains, fruits, and vegetables provide sustained energy levels, support cardiovascular health, and prevent blood sugar imbalances that can affect libido and erectile function.
- **Healthy Fats**: Omega-3 fatty acids found in fish, flaxseeds, chia seeds,

and walnuts promote cardiovascular health, reduce inflammation, and support hormone production critical for sexual function.

1. **Micronutrients**:

- **Zinc**: Zinc plays a crucial role in testosterone production, sperm health, and overall sexual function. Food sources rich in zinc include oysters, beef, pumpkin seeds, and legumes.
- **Vitamin D**: Adequate vitamin D levels are linked to improved testosterone levels, mood regulation, and bone health. Sources of vitamin D include sunlight exposure, fortified foods, fatty fish, and egg yolks.
- **Vitamin C**: Vitamin C is an antioxidant that supports blood vessel health, collagen production, and immune function. Citrus fruits, strawberries, bell peppers, and broccoli are excellent sources of vitamin C.
- **Vitamin E**: Vitamin E has antioxidant properties that protect cells from oxidative stress, potentially benefiting sexual health. Nuts, seeds, spinach, and avocado are rich in vitamin E.
- **Selenium**: Selenium is essential for sperm production and reproductive health. Brazil nuts, seafood, whole grains, and eggs are good sources of selenium.

Foods for Libido and Erectile Function

1. **Fruits and Vegetables**:

- **Berries**: Blueberries, strawberries, and raspberries are rich in antioxidants that support blood flow and cardiovascular health, important for erectile function.
- **Leafy Greens**: Spinach, kale, and Swiss chard provide nutrients like magnesium, folate, and vitamin C, which contribute to healthy blood circulation and hormone regulation.
- **Watermelon**: Contains citrulline, a compound that helps relax blood vessels and improve blood flow, potentially enhancing erectile function.

1. **Lean Proteins**:

- **Fish**: Fatty fish like salmon, mackerel, and sardines are high in omega-3 fatty acids, which promote heart health and may improve sexual function.
- **Poultry**: Chicken and turkey breast are lean protein sources that provide amino acids necessary for hormone production and muscle health.

1. **Nuts and Seeds**:

- **Almonds**: Rich in vitamin E and magnesium, almonds support cardiovascular health and may have positive effects on sexual function.
- **Pumpkin Seeds**: High in zinc, pumpkin seeds support testosterone production and sperm health, benefiting overall sexual health.

1. **Whole Grains**:

- **Oats**: Provide fiber, B vitamins, and minerals that support energy levels, hormone balance, and cardiovascular health, all of which are essential for sexual function.
- **Quinoa**: A nutrient-dense whole grain containing protein, fiber, and minerals like magnesium and zinc, supporting overall health and vitality.

Foods to Avoid or Limit

1. **Processed Foods**:

- **High-Sugar Foods**: Excessive sugar intake can contribute to insulin resistance, inflammation, and hormonal imbalances that may negatively impact sexual health.
- **Trans Fats**: Found in processed foods, fried foods, and some baked goods, trans fats can impair cardiovascular health and blood flow, affecting erectile function.

1. **Excessive Alcohol and Caffeine**:

- **Alcohol**: Heavy alcohol consumption can impair sexual function, decrease libido, and disrupt hormone production. Moderation is key to minimizing adverse effects.
- **Caffeine**: While moderate caffeine intake is generally safe, excessive caffeine consumption can lead to increased anxiety, disrupted sleep, and potential effects on sexual arousal.

1. **High-Sodium Foods**:

- **Processed Meats**: High-sodium processed meats like bacon, sausage, and deli meats can contribute to hypertension and cardiovascular issues, affecting sexual health.

Hydration and Sexual Health

Proper hydration is crucial for overall health, including sexual function. Adequate water intake supports blood circulation, nutrient transport, and hormone regulation, all of which are essential for optimal sexual health. Consuming water-rich foods such as fruits, vegetables, and herbal teas can contribute to hydration levels.

Dietary Supplements

While a balanced diet is the foundation of good nutrition, some individuals may benefit from dietary supplements that support sexual health. It's important to consult with a healthcare provider before starting any supplements. Some supplements that may be beneficial include:

1. **L-arginine**: An amino acid that supports blood vessel dilation and circulation, potentially improving erectile function.
2. **Ginseng**: Herbal supplement with potential benefits for libido, erectile

function, and overall vitality.

3. **Maca**: Root vegetable with traditional use for enhancing libido and sexual function.
4. **Fenugreek**: Herb known for its potential to support testosterone levels and sexual health.

Conclusion

Nutrition and diet play a significant role in male sexual health, influencing libido, erectile function, hormonal balance, and overall well-being. By incorporating nutrient-rich foods, prioritizing hydration, avoiding or limiting unhealthy choices, and considering supplements when appropriate, individuals can support optimal sexual function and enjoy a fulfilling and satisfying sex life. Consulting with healthcare professionals and nutrition experts can provide personalized guidance for addressing specific dietary needs and optimizing sexual health.

Four

Chapter 4: Exercise and Fitness

In this chapter, we will explore the profound impact of exercise and physical fitness on male sexual health. From improving cardiovascular function and hormone regulation to enhancing stamina and erectile function, regular physical activity plays a crucial role in maintaining optimal sexual well-being. We will delve into different types of exercises, their benefits for sexual health, and practical strategies for incorporating exercise into daily routines.

Benefits of Exercise for Sexual Health

1. **Cardiovascular Health**:

- **Improved Blood Flow**: Regular cardiovascular exercise, such as running, swimming, or cycling, promotes healthy blood circulation, including blood flow to the genital area. Enhanced blood flow can contribute to better erectile function and sexual arousal.
- **Heart Health**: Strong cardiovascular fitness reduces the risk of cardiovascular diseases, such as hypertension and atherosclerosis, which can impair sexual function.

1. **Hormone Regulation**:

- **Testosterone Levels**: Moderate to high-intensity exercise, combined with adequate rest and recovery, can support healthy testosterone levels, crucial for libido, muscle mass, and overall vitality.
- **Endorphin Release**: Exercise stimulates the release of endorphins, the body's natural feel-good hormones, which can enhance mood, reduce stress, and improve sexual desire.

1. **Stress Reduction**:

- **Stress Management**: Physical activity is a potent stress-reliever, helping to reduce cortisol levels and alleviate stress and anxiety. Lower stress levels can positively impact sexual function and satisfaction.

1. **Weight Management**:

- **Body Composition**: Maintaining a healthy weight through regular exercise and a balanced diet contributes to better body image, self-confidence, and sexual self-esteem.
- **Obesity and Sexual Health**: Obesity is linked to hormonal imbalances, reduced libido, erectile dysfunction, and other sexual health issues. Exercise plays a crucial role in preventing and managing obesity-related concerns.

Types of Exercise for Sexual Health

1. **Aerobic Exercise**:

- **Benefits**: Aerobic activities like brisk walking, jogging, dancing, and swimming improve cardiovascular fitness, enhance endurance, and promote overall well-being, all of which are beneficial for sexual health.
- **Frequency**: Aim for at least 150 minutes of moderate-intensity aerobic

exercise or 75 minutes of vigorous-intensity exercise per week, spread across multiple days.

1. **Strength Training**:

- **Benefits**: Resistance training with weights, resistance bands, or body-weight exercises strengthens muscles, boosts metabolism, and supports hormone production, including testosterone.
- **Focus Areas**: Include exercises targeting major muscle groups, such as squats, deadlifts, bench presses, and rows, to promote overall strength and functional fitness.

1. **Flexibility and Mobility**:

- **Benefits**: Stretching exercises, yoga, and mobility drills improve flexibility, joint range of motion, and posture, enhancing physical performance and reducing the risk of injuries during physical activity.
- **Incorporation**: Include stretching and mobility work as part of warm-ups, cool-downs, or dedicated flexibility sessions to maintain optimal movement patterns and prevent stiffness.

1. **Pelvic Floor Exercises**:

- **Benefits**: Strengthening the pelvic floor muscles through exercises like Kegels can improve erectile function, urinary control, and overall sexual satisfaction.
- **Technique**: Contract the pelvic floor muscles (the ones used to stop the flow of urine) for several seconds, then release. Gradually increase repetitions and hold times for progressive strengthening.

Strategies for Incorporating Exercise into Daily Life

1. **Set Realistic Goals**:

- **SMART Goals**: Create Specific, Measurable, Achievable, Relevant, and Time-bound goals related to exercise frequency, duration, and intensity. Start with manageable targets and gradually progress.

1. **Find Enjoyable Activities**:

- **Variety**: Explore different types of exercises to find activities you enjoy, whether it's jogging in nature, dancing to music, practicing yoga, or playing team sports. Enjoyable activities increase motivation and adherence to regular exercise.

1. **Schedule Regular Workouts**:

- **Consistency**: Establish a consistent exercise routine by scheduling workouts at convenient times during the week. Treat exercise as a priority, similar to other essential activities.

1. **Mix Cardio, Strength, and Flexibility**:

- **Balanced Approach**: Incorporate a combination of aerobic, strength training, and flexibility exercises to reap comprehensive benefits for physical fitness and sexual health.
- **Cross-Training**: Alternate between different types of workouts to prevent boredom, overuse injuries, and plateaus in fitness progress.

1. **Include Partner Activities**:

- **Couples Workouts**: Engaging in physical activities with a partner, such as partner yoga, dancing, or outdoor sports, can foster bonding, enhance motivation, and make exercise more enjoyable.

1. **Prioritize Recovery**:

- **Rest Days**: Include rest days in your exercise routine to allow for adequate recovery and muscle repair. Listen to your body's signals and avoid overtraining, which can lead to fatigue and burnout.

1. **Consult with Professionals**:

- **Fitness Experts**: Consider consulting with fitness professionals, such as personal trainers or physical therapists, to design personalized exercise programs, learn proper techniques, and receive guidance on injury prevention.

Exercise and Sexual Performance

Regular exercise not only benefits overall health and well-being but also contributes to improved sexual performance and satisfaction. Some ways exercise can positively impact sexual performance include:

1. **Enhanced Stamina**: Improved cardiovascular fitness and endurance from regular exercise can lead to longer-lasting sexual activity and increased stamina.
2. **Increased Blood Flow**: Aerobic exercise promotes healthy blood circulation, including to the genital area, supporting erectile function and arousal.
3. **Improved Body Confidence**: Regular exercise and fitness improvements can boost self-confidence, body image, and sexual self-esteem, enhancing sexual performance and enjoyment.
4. **Stress Reduction**: Exercise helps reduce stress, anxiety, and tension, creating a more relaxed and enjoyable environment for sexual activity.
5. **Hormone Regulation**: Physical activity supports hormonal balance,

including testosterone levels, which can positively influence libido, erectile function, and overall sexual health.

Conclusion

Exercise and physical fitness are integral components of male sexual health, offering numerous benefits for libido, erectile function, hormone regulation, cardiovascular health, stress management, and overall well-being. By incorporating a balanced mix of aerobic, strength training, flexibility, and pelvic floor exercises into regular routines, individuals can optimize their sexual health, performance, and satisfaction. Consistency, enjoyment, realistic goal-setting, and proper recovery are key principles for successful integration of exercise into daily life. Consulting with fitness professionals and healthcare providers can provide personalized guidance and support for achieving fitness and sexual health goals.

Five

Chapter 5: Sleep and Rest

This chapter explores the critical role of sleep and rest in male sexual health and overall well-being. Adequate sleep duration and quality are essential for hormone regulation, energy levels, cognitive function, mood stability, and immune system function. We will delve into the impact of sleep on libido, erectile function, testosterone levels, and strategies for improving sleep hygiene to support optimal sexual health.

The Importance of Sleep for Sexual Health

1. **Hormone Regulation**:

- **Testosterone Production**: Sleep plays a crucial role in testosterone synthesis and release. Adequate sleep duration, particularly during deep sleep stages, supports healthy testosterone levels, essential for libido, muscle mass, and reproductive function.
- **Growth Hormone Release**: Deep sleep phases also stimulate the release of growth hormone, which contributes to tissue repair, muscle growth, and overall vitality.

1. **Libido and Sexual Desire**:

- **Sleep Quality and Libido**: Poor sleep quality, inadequate sleep duration, or sleep disturbances can lead to reduced libido, decreased sexual desire, and diminished sexual satisfaction.
- **Mood and Stress**: Quality sleep promotes emotional stability, reduces stress levels, and enhances mood, all of which are critical for sexual well-being and intimacy.

1. **Erectile Function**:

- **Nocturnal Erections**: During REM (rapid eye movement) sleep, men often experience spontaneous erections, known as nocturnal penile tumescence (NPT). These nocturnal erections contribute to erectile health, penile tissue oxygenation, and maintenance of erectile function.
- **Sleep Disorders and Erectile Dysfunction (ED)**: Sleep disorders like sleep apnea, insomnia, or restless leg syndrome can contribute to erectile dysfunction by disrupting sleep patterns, reducing oxygen levels, and impacting hormone regulation.

1. **Energy Levels and Stamina**:

- **Restorative Sleep**: Quality sleep is essential for physical and mental recovery, replenishing energy stores, and supporting stamina and endurance, which are vital for sexual activity and performance.

Strategies for Improving Sleep Hygiene

1. **Consistent Sleep Schedule**:

- **Bedtime Routine**: Establish a consistent bedtime routine to signal to your body that it's time to wind down and prepare for sleep. Consistency helps regulate the internal body clock (circadian rhythm) and promotes

better sleep quality.
- **Wake-Up Time**: Aim to wake up at the same time each day, even on weekends, to maintain a regular sleep-wake cycle.

1. **Create a Sleep-Conducive Environment**:

- **Darkness and Quietness**: Keep your bedroom dark, quiet, and comfortable to minimize disruptions and promote relaxation. Consider using blackout curtains, white noise machines, or earplugs if needed.
- **Comfortable Bedding**: Invest in a comfortable mattress, pillows, and bedding that support proper alignment and promote restful sleep.

1. **Limit Screen Time Before Bed**:

- **Blue Light Exposure**: Reduce exposure to blue light from electronic devices (phones, tablets, computers, TVs) in the hour leading up to bedtime. Blue light can suppress melatonin production, a hormone crucial for sleep regulation.
- **Night Mode or Blue Light Filters**: Use night mode settings or blue light filtering apps on devices to reduce blue light emission during nighttime use.

1. **Mindful Relaxation Techniques**:

- **Deep Breathing**: Practice deep breathing exercises, such as diaphragmatic breathing or progressive muscle relaxation, to promote relaxation and reduce stress before bedtime.
- **Mindfulness Meditation**: Engage in mindfulness meditation or guided relaxation techniques to calm the mind, release tension, and improve sleep quality.

1. **Limit Stimulants and Alcohol**:

- **Caffeine**: Avoid consuming caffeine-containing beverages (coffee, tea, energy drinks) in the afternoon and evening, as caffeine can interfere with sleep onset and quality.
- **Alcohol**: While alcohol may initially induce drowsiness, it can disrupt sleep cycles, lead to fragmented sleep, and worsen sleep apnea symptoms. Limit alcohol consumption, especially close to bedtime.

1. **Regular Exercise**:

- **Timing**: Engage in regular physical activity, but avoid vigorous exercise close to bedtime, as it may increase alertness and delay sleep onset. Moderate exercise earlier in the day can promote better sleep quality.
- **Benefits**: Regular exercise contributes to overall health, reduces stress, and improves sleep quality, indirectly benefiting sexual health and well-being.

1. **Healthy Sleep Habits**:

- **Avoid Napping Late**: Limit daytime naps and avoid napping late in the day, as it can interfere with nighttime sleep.
- **Limit Fluid Intake**: Reduce fluid intake close to bedtime to minimize disruptions from nocturnal urination.
- **Comfortable Temperature**: Maintain a comfortable room temperature for sleep, as extreme temperatures can disrupt sleep quality.

Addressing Sleep Disorders

If you experience persistent sleep difficulties or suspect a sleep disorder, it's essential to seek evaluation and management from healthcare professionals, such as sleep specialists or primary care providers. Common sleep disorders that can impact sexual health include:

1. **Sleep Apnea**:

- **Symptoms**: Loud snoring, gasping or choking during sleep, daytime fatigue, and irritability.
- **Impact on Sexual Health**: Sleep apnea can lead to decreased oxygen levels, fragmented sleep, and hormonal imbalances, contributing to erectile dysfunction and reduced libido.

1. **Insomnia**:

- **Symptoms**: Difficulty falling asleep, staying asleep, or waking up too early, leading to daytime fatigue and impaired functioning.
- **Impact on Sexual Health**: Insomnia can cause sleep deprivation, mood disturbances, and reduced libido, affecting sexual desire and satisfaction.

1. **Restless Leg Syndrome (RLS)**:

- **Symptoms**: Uncomfortable sensations in the legs, often accompanied by an urge to move the legs, especially at night.
- **Impact on Sexual Health**: RLS-related sleep disturbances can disrupt sleep quality, lead to daytime sleepiness, and impact sexual function and well-being.

Conclusion

Sleep and rest are foundational pillars of male sexual health, influencing libido, erectile function, hormone regulation, energy levels, and overall well-being. By prioritizing good sleep hygiene, creating a sleep-conducive environment, managing stress, and seeking evaluation and treatment for sleep disorders when needed, individuals can optimize their sleep quality and support optimal sexual health and satisfaction. Consistency, mindfulness, and healthy sleep habits are key to fostering restorative sleep and enhancing overall quality of life.

Chapter 6: Lifestyle Habits

In this chapter, we'll explore the impact of lifestyle habits on male sexual health. Lifestyle choices, including smoking, alcohol consumption, drug use, and overall wellness practices, can significantly influence libido, erectile function, hormone balance, and overall sexual well-being. Understanding the role of lifestyle habits and adopting healthy behaviors can promote optimal sexual health and satisfaction.

Smoking and Sexual Health

1. **Impact on Blood Flow:**

- Smoking damages blood vessels and reduces blood flow throughout the body, including to the genital area. This can lead to erectile dysfunction (ED) or contribute to existing ED issues.
- Nicotine constricts blood vessels, limiting the ability to achieve and maintain erections.

1. **Hormonal Imbalance:**

- Smoking can disrupt hormone balance, including testosterone levels. Reduced testosterone can affect libido and sexual performance.

1. **Sperm Quality**:

- Smoking is associated with decreased sperm quality, including lower sperm count, motility, and morphology, which can impact fertility and reproductive health.

Alcohol Consumption and Sexual Function

1. **Immediate Effects**:

- While moderate alcohol consumption may lower inhibitions and enhance arousal initially, excessive alcohol intake can lead to impaired sexual performance, including difficulty achieving or maintaining erections.
- Chronic alcohol abuse can contribute to long-term sexual health issues, including decreased libido, hormonal imbalances, and erectile dysfunction.

1. **Interference with Hormones**:

- Alcohol can interfere with hormone production and regulation, including testosterone levels, which are crucial for sexual desire and function.

Drug Use and Sexual Health

1. **Illegal Drugs**:

- Recreational drug use, including substances like cocaine, heroin, or methamphetamines, can have detrimental effects on sexual health. These drugs can impair sexual function, decrease libido, and lead to addiction, impacting overall well-being.

- Injection drug use also poses risks such as increased susceptibility to infections, which can affect sexual health and fertility.

1. **Medication Abuse**:

- Misuse or abuse of prescription medications, particularly those that affect the central nervous system or hormone levels, can lead to sexual health issues such as erectile dysfunction, decreased libido, or hormonal imbalances.

Healthy Lifestyle Practices for Sexual Health

1. **Regular Physical Activity**:

- Engaging in regular exercise promotes cardiovascular health, improves blood flow, supports hormone regulation, and enhances overall well-being, all of which benefit sexual health and function.

1. **Balanced Dict**:

- Consuming a nutritious diet rich in fruits, vegetables, lean proteins, whole grains, and healthy fats provides essential nutrients for sexual health, hormone production, and energy levels.
- Limiting processed foods, sugar, and excessive salt intake can also support overall wellness and sexual function.

1. **Stress Management**:

- Chronic stress can negatively impact sexual health by increasing cortisol levels, affecting hormone balance, and reducing libido. Practicing stress-reduction techniques such as mindfulness, meditation, deep breathing, and regular physical activity can promote relaxation and improve sexual well-being.

1. **Adequate Sleep**:

- Prioritizing quality sleep is crucial for hormone regulation, energy levels, mood stability, and overall health. Adequate rest supports sexual function and satisfaction.

1. **Hydration**:

- Staying hydrated is essential for overall health, including sexual function. Drinking enough water supports circulation, nutrient transport, and cellular function, contributing to optimal sexual health.

1. **Avoiding Risky Behaviors**:

- Engaging in safe sex practices, avoiding multiple sexual partners without protection, and getting regular sexual health screenings can prevent sexually transmitted infections (STIs) and promote sexual well-being.

Seeking Professional Help

1. **Smoking Cessation Programs**:

- For individuals struggling with nicotine addiction, smoking cessation programs, support groups, counseling, and nicotine replacement therapies (such as patches or gums) can help quit smoking and improve overall health.

1. **Alcohol and Drug Rehabilitation**:

- For individuals dealing with alcohol or drug dependency, seeking professional rehabilitation programs, counseling, and support groups can aid in recovery and promote healthier lifestyle choices.

1. **Behavioral Therapy**:

- Behavioral therapy, counseling, or sex therapy can address underlying psychological factors contributing to sexual health issues and help develop healthier attitudes and behaviors related to sex and intimacy.

Conclusion

Lifestyle habits profoundly impact male sexual health, including libido, erectile function, hormone balance, and overall well-being. Adopting healthy lifestyle practices such as regular physical activity, balanced nutrition, stress management, adequate sleep, hydration, and avoiding risky behaviors can promote optimal sexual function and satisfaction. Seeking professional help when needed, such as smoking cessation programs, rehabilitation for substance abuse, or therapy for psychological factors, can support positive changes and enhance overall quality of life. Prioritizing health-conscious choices and addressing harmful habits can contribute to a fulfilling and satisfying sex life.

Seven

Chapter 7: Communication and Intimacy

This chapter delves into the pivotal role of communication and intimacy in fostering healthy relationships and promoting sexual well-being for males. Effective communication, emotional connection, and intimacy are essential elements that contribute to a fulfilling and satisfying sex life. We'll explore the importance of open communication, emotional vulnerability, trust, and intimacy-building practices for enhancing relationships and sexual satisfaction.

Importance of Communication in Relationships

1. **Establishing Trust:**

- Open and honest communication builds trust and fosters emotional intimacy between partners. Trust is essential for creating a safe and supportive environment for sexual exploration and expression.

1. **Expressing Needs and Desires**:

- Effective communication allows individuals to express their sexual needs, desires, boundaries, and preferences openly and without judgment. This clarity promotes understanding and mutual satisfaction in sexual encounters.

1. **Addressing Concerns and Challenges**:

- Communication enables partners to address sexual concerns, challenges, or issues that may arise, such as erectile dysfunction, low libido, performance anxiety, or changes in sexual interests over time. By discussing these matters openly, couples can seek solutions together and strengthen their connection.

1. **Enhancing Emotional Intimacy**:

- Meaningful conversations, shared experiences, and emotional support contribute to deepening emotional intimacy, which is a foundation for satisfying sexual relationships.

Effective Communication Strategies

1. **Active Listening**:

- Practice active listening by giving your partner your full attention, maintaining eye contact, and validating their feelings and experiences. Avoid interrupting or dismissing their thoughts and emotions.
- Reflective listening techniques, such as paraphrasing what your partner has said to ensure understanding, can enhance communication effectiveness.

1. **Nonverbal Communication**:

- Pay attention to nonverbal cues, such as body language, facial expressions, and tone of voice, as they can convey emotions and messages that complement verbal communication.

- Nonverbal gestures of affection, such as hugs, kisses, holding hands, or gentle touch, can strengthen emotional bonds and intimacy.

1. **Use "I" Statements**:

- Express thoughts, feelings, and concerns using "I" statements to take ownership of your emotions and avoid blaming or accusing language. For example, "I feel disconnected when we don't spend quality time together" conveys personal feelings without placing blame.

1. **Be Respectful and Empathetic**:

- Respect your partner's perspectives, boundaries, and preferences, even if they differ from your own. Practice empathy by trying to understand their feelings and experiences from their point of view.
- Avoid judgment, criticism, or defensiveness during discussions about sensitive topics, including sexual matters.

Sexual Communication and Exploration

1. **Initiating Conversations**:

- Initiate discussions about sexual desires, fantasies, boundaries, and expectations in a non-threatening and respectful manner. Create a safe space where both partners feel comfortable expressing their thoughts and needs.
- Regularly check in with each other about sexual satisfaction, changes in desires or preferences, and any concerns or issues that may arise.

1. **Exploring Together**:

- Explore new sexual experiences, activities, or fantasies together with mutual consent and enthusiasm. Communicate openly about likes, dislikes, and any adjustments needed to enhance pleasure and intimacy.

- Experimentation and variety can add excitement and novelty to the relationship, contributing to sexual satisfaction.

1. **Seeking Professional Guidance**:

- If sexual concerns or challenges persist despite open communication and efforts to address them, consider seeking guidance from a qualified sex therapist or counselor. Professional support can offer valuable insights, strategies, and interventions for improving sexual health and intimacy.

Building Emotional Intimacy

1. **Emotional Connection**:

- Engage in meaningful conversations, share personal experiences, thoughts, and feelings, and actively listen to each other to deepen emotional connection and understanding.
- Express appreciation, affection, and gratitude regularly to strengthen emotional bonds and foster a positive relationship dynamic.

1. **Quality Time Together**:

- Prioritize quality time together without distractions, such as phones or work-related activities. Engage in activities that promote bonding, laughter, and shared experiences, reinforcing emotional intimacy.
- Plan date nights, outings, or activities that you both enjoy to nurture the relationship outside of daily responsibilities.

1. **Vulnerability and Trust**:

- Be vulnerable with your partner by sharing fears, insecurities, and vulnerabilities in a supportive and non-judgmental environment. Building trust through vulnerability enhances emotional intimacy and strengthens the relationship.

Addressing Relationship Challenges

1. **Conflict Resolution**:

- Develop healthy conflict resolution skills by practicing active listening, empathy, compromise, and finding mutually beneficial solutions to disagreements or misunderstandings.
- Avoiding unresolved conflicts or recurring arguments can create barriers to intimacy and communication.

1. **Seeking Support**:

- If relationship challenges or conflicts persist, consider seeking couples counseling or therapy to address underlying issues, improve communication, and rebuild relationship harmony.
- Professional guidance can provide valuable tools, strategies, and insights for navigating relationship challenges and fostering a healthy, fulfilling partnership.

Conclusion

Effective communication and emotional intimacy are foundational pillars of healthy relationships and satisfying sexual experiences. By prioritizing open and honest communication, active listening, empathy, and vulnerability, couples can enhance their emotional connection, trust, and sexual satisfaction. Regularly discussing sexual desires, boundaries, and concerns, exploring new experiences together, and seeking professional support when needed can strengthen relationships and promote lifelong intimacy and well-being. Cultivating a supportive and communicative partnership enriches both emotional and sexual aspects of the relationship, fostering mutual growth and fulfillment.

Eight

Chapter 8: Techniques for Longer Lasting Sex

This chapter delves into various techniques and strategies aimed at prolonging sexual activity and enhancing sexual satisfaction for males. Longer-lasting sex can lead to increased pleasure, intimacy, and overall sexual well-being. We'll explore techniques for improving stamina, managing arousal levels, and promoting mutual pleasure in sexual encounters.

Understanding Ejaculation Control

1. **Start-Stop Technique**:

- This technique involves pausing sexual stimulation (such as penetration or manual stimulation) when nearing ejaculation. Take a short break to allow arousal levels to decrease before resuming activity.
- By practicing this technique, individuals can gain better control over their arousal and delay ejaculation, leading to longer-lasting sexual experiences.

1. **Squeeze Technique**:

- During the squeeze technique, the base of the penis is gently squeezed for several seconds when nearing ejaculation. This action can reduce arousal and delay ejaculation.
- Communication with your partner is crucial when using this technique to ensure comfort and mutual understanding.

Breathing and Relaxation Techniques

1. **Deep Breathing**:

- Deep, slow breathing can help reduce anxiety, tension, and arousal levels during sexual activity. Focus on diaphragmatic breathing, inhaling deeply through the nose and exhaling slowly through the mouth.
- Incorporate deep breathing exercises into foreplay and sexual encounters to promote relaxation and prolongation of sexual activity.

1. **Progressive Muscle Relaxation**:

- Progressive muscle relaxation involves tensing and then releasing different muscle groups throughout the body, starting from the toes and working up to the head.
- This technique promotes overall relaxation, reduces muscle tension, and can aid in delaying ejaculation by managing arousal levels.

Pelvic Floor Exercises

1. **Kegel Exercises**:

- Kegel exercises strengthen the pelvic floor muscles, which play a role in ejaculation control and erectile function.
- To perform Kegels, contract the pelvic floor muscles (the ones used to stop urine flow) and hold for several seconds before releasing. Gradually increase repetitions and hold times for improved muscle strength and

control.

Sensate Focus and Mindfulness

1. **Sensate Focus**:

- Sensate focus exercises involve non-genital touching and exploration of each other's bodies to enhance sensory awareness, arousal, and intimacy without the pressure of orgasm.
- By focusing on sensory experiences and pleasure rather than performance or ejaculation, couples can prolong sexual activity and deepen emotional connection.

1. **Mindfulness Practices**:

- Mindfulness techniques, such as mindfulness meditation or guided imagery, can help individuals stay present and focused during sexual activity, reducing performance anxiety and enhancing enjoyment.
- Mindful awareness of sensations, emotions, and breathing patterns can contribute to longer-lasting and more satisfying sexual experiences.

Communication and Mutual Pleasure

1. **Communication About Preferences**:

- Open communication with your partner about sexual preferences, desires, and boundaries can lead to more satisfying and mutually pleasurable sexual encounters.
- Discussing expectations, fantasies, and ways to enhance pleasure can create a supportive and enjoyable sexual environment.

1. **Mutual Stimulation**:

- Incorporate mutual stimulation, such as manual stimulation or oral sex, into sexual activities to prolong arousal and pleasure for both partners.
- Explore erogenous zones, experiment with different techniques, and prioritize mutual satisfaction and enjoyment.

Delay Sprays and Condoms

1. **Delay Sprays**:

- Over-the-counter delay sprays or creams containing mild anesthetics (such as lidocaine or benzocaine) can help reduce penile sensitivity and delay ejaculation.
- Follow product instructions carefully and communicate with your partner about using such products for mutual comfort and satisfaction.

1. **Thicker Condoms**:

- Using thicker condoms or those designed for extended pleasure can reduce penile sensitivity and prolong sexual activity.
- Experiment with different condom types and brands to find one that enhances pleasure while providing adequate protection.

Mental Techniques and Distraction Methods

1. **Mental Distraction**:

- Engaging in mental distraction techniques, such as focusing on non-sexual thoughts or activities during moments of intense arousal, can help delay ejaculation.
- Redirecting attention away from sexual stimulation temporarily can reduce arousal levels and prolong sexual activity.

1. **Fantasy Exploration**:

- Exploring erotic fantasies or role-playing scenarios can enhance arousal and prolong sexual excitement, leading to longer-lasting sexual encounters.
- Communication with your partner about shared fantasies or preferences is essential for mutual enjoyment and consent.

Conclusion

Techniques for longer-lasting sex encompass a range of strategies focused on ejaculation control, arousal management, relaxation, communication, and mutual pleasure. By incorporating these techniques into sexual encounters, individuals and couples can prolong arousal, delay ejaculation, enhance intimacy, and promote overall sexual satisfaction. Experimentation, open communication, mutual exploration, and mindfulness during sexual activities contribute to a fulfilling and enjoyable sex life. It's important to remember that sexual preferences and needs vary among individuals, so finding what works best for you and your partner through experimentation and communication is key to a satisfying sexual experience.

Nine

Chapter 9: Understanding Libido

Libido, often referred to as sex drive or sexual desire, plays a significant role in the sexual health and well-being of males. This chapter aims to delve into the complex nature of libido, exploring its various factors, influences, and strategies for maintaining a healthy and satisfying sex drive.

What is Libido?

Libido encompasses an individual's overall sexual desire and interest in sexual activity. It involves psychological, physiological, and hormonal factors that influence sexual arousal and motivation. Understanding libido involves exploring its components and how they interact to shape sexual desires and behaviors.

Factors Influencing Libido

1. **Hormonal Balance**:

- Testosterone: Testosterone levels play a crucial role in male libido. Adequate testosterone production supports healthy sexual desire, arousal, and erectile function. Hormonal imbalances, such as low testosterone levels, can lead to decreased libido.

- Other Hormones: Hormones like dopamine, estrogen, progesterone, and oxytocin also contribute to libido regulation and sexual arousal.

1. **Psychological Factors**:

- Stress and Anxiety: High levels of stress, anxiety, or mental health conditions like depression can negatively impact libido. Addressing psychological well-being is essential for maintaining healthy sexual desire.
- Relationship Dynamics: The quality of relationships, emotional connection, communication, trust, and intimacy with a partner can influence libido levels. Positive relationships often correlate with higher sexual desire.
- Body Image and Self-Esteem: Body image issues, low self-esteem, and confidence issues can affect sexual confidence and libido. Cultivating a positive self-image and addressing self-esteem concerns can improve sexual desire.

1. **Lifestyle and Health**:

- Physical Health: Overall physical health, including cardiovascular health, weight management, and chronic health conditions, can impact libido. Maintaining a healthy lifestyle through regular exercise, balanced nutrition, and adequate sleep supports sexual well-being.
- Substance Use: Excessive alcohol consumption, smoking, recreational drug use, and certain medications can affect libido negatively. Moderation and healthy lifestyle choices are essential.
- Fatigue and Sleep Quality: Fatigue, sleep disturbances, and sleep disorders can reduce energy levels and libido. Prioritizing restful sleep and managing fatigue are crucial for sexual health.

1. **Age and Hormonal Changes**:

- Aging: Libido can fluctuate with age due to changes in hormone production, metabolism, and physical health. While some individuals experience decreased libido as they age, others maintain healthy sexual desire with proper lifestyle habits and hormonal balance.

Strategies for Maintaining Healthy Libido

1. **Hormone Regulation**:

- Testosterone Levels: Regular physical activity, a balanced diet, adequate sleep, and stress management contribute to healthy testosterone levels. Consultation with healthcare providers may be necessary for addressing hormonal imbalances.
- Medication Review: Some medications, such as antidepressants or certain blood pressure medications, can affect libido. Discussing medication-related side effects with healthcare providers and exploring alternatives may be beneficial.

1. **Stress Management**:

- Stress Reduction Techniques: Engage in stress-relief activities such as meditation, deep breathing exercises, yoga, mindfulness practices, or hobbies to manage stress levels effectively.
- Work-Life Balance: Strive for a healthy work-life balance, set realistic goals, prioritize self-care, and establish boundaries to reduce stress and support overall well-being.

1. **Healthy Lifestyle Habits**:

- Balanced Nutrition: Consume a diet rich in fruits, vegetables, lean proteins, whole grains, and healthy fats. Avoid excessive sugar, processed foods, and alcohol, which can negatively impact libido and overall health.

- Regular Exercise: Engage in regular physical activity, including aerobic exercise, strength training, and flexibility exercises, to promote cardiovascular health, hormone regulation, and overall well-being.
- Quality Sleep: Prioritize adequate sleep duration and quality to support hormone production, energy levels, and overall vitality.

1. **Relationship Enhancement**:

- Communication and Intimacy: Foster open communication, emotional connection, trust, and intimacy in relationships. Discuss sexual desires, preferences, concerns, and explore ways to enhance sexual satisfaction together.
- Relationship Counseling: If relationship issues or communication barriers affect libido, consider couples counseling or therapy to address underlying concerns and strengthen the relationship.

1. **Mental and Emotional Well-Being**:

- Address Mental Health: Seek support and treatment for mental health conditions such as depression, anxiety, or stress-related disorders. Psychotherapy, counseling, or medication may be beneficial in managing psychological factors that impact libido.
- Self-Care Practices: Practice self-care, relaxation techniques, hobbies, and activities that promote emotional well-being, reduce stress, and enhance overall life satisfaction.

Libido and Aging

1. **Understanding Age-Related Changes**:

- Hormonal Shifts: Aging is associated with natural changes in hormone production, including testosterone decline in males. These hormonal shifts can influence libido and sexual function.

- Physical Health: Age-related health conditions, medication use, and lifestyle factors can affect libido. Managing chronic health conditions, staying active, and maintaining a healthy lifestyle are crucial for sexual health as individuals age.

1. **Adapting Sexual Expectations**:

- Open Communication: Discuss sexual expectations, desires, and concerns openly with your partner, especially as you navigate age-related changes. Adjusting sexual activities, exploring new techniques, and prioritizing intimacy can enhance sexual satisfaction.
- Professional Guidance: Consult healthcare providers or sexual health specialists for guidance on managing age-related sexual changes, addressing erectile dysfunction, and maintaining a fulfilling sex life.

Conclusion

Libido is a multifaceted aspect of male sexual health influenced by hormonal, psychological, lifestyle, and relational factors. Maintaining a healthy libido involves addressing hormonal balance, managing stress, adopting healthy lifestyle habits, nurturing relationships, and prioritizing mental and emotional well-being. Understanding individual variations in libido and seeking appropriate support when needed contribute to a fulfilling and satisfying sex life across different life stages. Open communication, self-awareness, and proactive health management are key elements in promoting healthy libido and sexual well-being.

Ten

Chapter 10: Sexual Fantasies and Exploration

This chapter delves into the realm of sexual fantasies and exploration, emphasizing their role in enhancing sexual arousal, intimacy, and satisfaction for males. Understanding and embracing sexual fantasies, exploring new experiences, and fostering open communication with partners can contribute to a fulfilling and dynamic sex life.

Understanding Sexual Fantasies

1. **Definition of Sexual Fantasies**:

- Sexual fantasies are mental images, scenarios, or thoughts that elicit sexual arousal and desire. They can range from simple fantasies to elaborate scenarios involving various themes, desires, or experiences.
- Fantasies are a natural part of human sexuality and can enhance arousal, creativity, and sexual satisfaction.

1. **Role of Fantasies in Sexual Arousal**:

- Fantasies often play a significant role in sexual arousal, acting as a catalyst for desire and excitement. They can stimulate the imagination, enhance pleasure, and contribute to a more satisfying sexual experience.

- Fantasies allow individuals to explore desires, preferences, and fantasies that may not be feasible or practical in reality, providing a safe space for sexual exploration and expression.

Types of Sexual Fantasies

1. **Erotic Fantasies**:

- Erotic fantasies involve scenarios or images of sexual encounters, fantasies, or activities that elicit arousal and excitement. They can range from romantic and sensual to more adventurous or taboo themes.
- Examples include fantasizing about specific sexual acts, locations, partners, role-playing scenarios, or exploring different fantasies to enhance arousal and pleasure.

1. **Emotional Fantasies**:

- Emotional fantasies focus on emotional connections, intimacy, and romantic scenarios rather than explicit sexual acts. They may involve feelings of love, passion, connection, or emotional fulfillment.
- Emotional fantasies can deepen emotional intimacy, enhance sexual bonding, and contribute to overall relationship satisfaction.

1. **Power Dynamics and BDSM Fantasies**:

- Some individuals may have fantasies involving power dynamics, dominance, submission, bondage, discipline, or sadomasochism (BDSM). These fantasies can be consensual, negotiated, and explored safely within a trusting relationship.
- Communication, consent, and understanding boundaries are crucial when exploring BDSM or power-play fantasies to ensure mutual satis-

faction and safety.

1. **Taboo or Forbidden Fantasies**:

- Taboo fantasies involve desires or scenarios considered socially or culturally taboo, such as exhibitionism, voyeurism, incest fantasies, or age-play fantasies. It's important to note that fantasy does not equate to real-life actions, and consensual fantasy exploration is distinct from harmful behaviors.
- Fantasy exploration allows individuals to explore and understand their desires, boundaries, and fantasies without judgment or shame.

Benefits of Sexual Fantasies and Exploration

1. **Enhanced Arousal and Excitement**:

- Sexual fantasies can enhance arousal, excitement, and sexual anticipation, leading to more intense and satisfying sexual experiences.
- Exploring new fantasies or incorporating fantasies into sexual activities can add novelty, creativity, and excitement to the bedroom.

1. **Self-Discovery and Exploration**:

- Fantasies provide a platform for self-discovery, exploring desires, preferences, and boundaries. They can help individuals understand their sexual identity, interests, and erotic triggers.
- Fantasy exploration encourages curiosity, self-expression, and sexual confidence, contributing to a positive sexual self-image.

1. **Intimacy and Connection**:

- Sharing fantasies with a partner fosters open communication, trust, and intimacy. It allows couples to connect on a deeper level, understand each other's desires, and explore mutual fantasies together.

- Mutual exploration of fantasies can strengthen emotional bonds, enhance sexual compatibility, and promote relationship satisfaction.

Communication About Fantasies

1. **Creating a Safe and Non-Judgmental Space**:

- Foster open communication with your partner about sexual fantasies in a safe, non-judgmental environment. Encourage honesty, mutual respect, and understanding when discussing fantasies.
- Emphasize that fantasies are a normal and healthy part of sexuality, and exploring fantasies does not imply dissatisfaction with the current relationship or partner.

1. **Sharing Fantasies and Desires**:

- Share your fantasies, desires, and interests with your partner, and encourage them to do the same. Discuss boundaries, preferences, and any concerns openly to ensure mutual comfort and consent.
- Respect each other's boundaries, and prioritize consent and communication during fantasy exploration or role-playing scenarios.

Fantasy Exploration Techniques

1. **Role-Playing**:

- Engage in role-playing scenarios based on shared fantasies or interests. Role-playing allows couples to embody different roles, characters, or scenarios, adding excitement and novelty to sexual encounters.
- Communicate about roles, boundaries, and expectations beforehand to ensure a positive and consensual experience.

1. **Erotic Literature and Media**:

- Explore erotic literature, movies, or media that align with your fantasies or interests. Reading erotic stories or watching sensual content together can spark discussions, ignite arousal, and inspire new fantasies.
- Discuss reactions, fantasies, and preferences prompted by erotic content to deepen intimacy and understanding.

1. **Fantasy Fulfillment**:

- Consider ways to incorporate elements of fantasies into sexual activities, such as using props, costumes, role-playing scenarios, or trying new positions or activities that align with fantasy themes.
- Prioritize consent, communication, and mutual pleasure when exploring fantasy fulfillment to ensure a positive and enjoyable experience for both partners.

Managing Expectations and Boundaries

1. **Realism vs. Fantasy**:

- Differentiate between fantasy scenarios and real-life expectations. Understand that fantasies may not always translate into practical or feasible experiences, and that's okay.
- Communicate about boundaries, comfort levels, and realistic expectations when exploring fantasies to ensure a positive and respectful experience.

1. **Consent and Mutual Satisfaction**:

- Prioritize consent, mutual satisfaction, and emotional safety when exploring fantasies or engaging in fantasy fulfillment activities. Respect each other's boundaries, preferences, and comfort levels at all times.

- Check in with your partner during and after fantasy exploration to ensure mutual satisfaction, address any concerns, and maintain open communication.

Conclusion

Sexual fantasies and exploration play a vital role in sexual arousal, intimacy, and satisfaction for males. Understanding, embracing, and communicating about fantasies can enhance sexual excitement, deepen emotional connections, and promote mutual satisfaction in relationships. By creating a safe, non-judgmental space for fantasy exploration, fostering open communication, and respecting boundaries and consent, individuals and couples can enrich their sexual experiences and discover new dimensions of pleasure and intimacy. Fantasy exploration encourages curiosity, creativity, and self-expression, contributing to a fulfilling and dynamic sex life.

Eleven

Chapter 11: Sexual Positions and Techniques

This chapter delves into the world of sexual positions and techniques, exploring a variety of ways to enhance pleasure, intimacy, and satisfaction during sexual encounters for males. Understanding different positions, techniques, and tips can contribute to a more fulfilling and enjoyable sex life.

Importance of Sexual Positions and Techniques

1. **Enhanced Physical Pleasure:**

- Different sexual positions and techniques can stimulate erogenous zones, increase friction, and target sensitive areas, enhancing physical pleasure and arousal for both partners.
- Exploring a variety of positions allows individuals and couples to discover what works best for their unique preferences, anatomy, and desires.

1. **Variety and Novelty:**

- Incorporating different positions and techniques adds variety, excitement, and novelty to sexual experiences, preventing routine and monotony.

- Trying new positions or techniques can reignite passion, curiosity, and exploration in the bedroom, keeping sexual encounters engaging and fulfilling.

1. **Emotional Connection**:

- Certain positions and techniques promote intimate eye contact, physical closeness, and emotional connection between partners, enhancing intimacy and bonding.
- Communication, trust, and mutual pleasure are key elements in exploring sexual positions and techniques to create a positive and satisfying experience.

Exploring Sexual Positions

1. **Missionary Position**:

- The missionary position involves the penetrating partner on top, with the receiving partner lying on their back. This position allows for deep penetration, intimate eye contact, and easy access to erogenous zones.
- Variations: Experiment with leg positions, angles, or adding pillows for support and comfort. Placing a pillow under the receiving partner's hips can enhance sensation and allow for better G-spot or prostate stimulation.

1. **Doggy Style**:

- In the doggy style position, the penetrating partner enters from behind while the receiving partner is on hands and knees or leaning forward. This position offers deeper penetration, access to erogenous zones, and a sense of dominance or submission.
- Variations: Try different angles, such as adjusting the height or positioning of the receiving partner, or incorporating manual stimulation of

erogenous zones for added pleasure.

1. **Cowgirl/Reverse Cowgirl**:

- The cowgirl position involves the receiving partner straddling the penetrating partner, facing them (cowgirl) or facing away (reverse cowgirl). This position allows the receiving partner control over depth, pace, and angle of penetration.
- Variations: Experiment with rocking, grinding, or bouncing motions, and adjust the angle for optimal clitoral or penile stimulation. Reverse cowgirl offers a view of the receiving partner's backside, adding visual excitement.

1. **Spooning**:

- Spooning involves both partners lying on their sides, with the penetrating partner entering from behind. This position promotes closeness, intimacy, and deep penetration while allowing for relaxed and comfortable positioning.
- Variations: Adjust the angle by raising or lowering the top leg, or incorporating manual stimulation of erogenous zones such as breasts, nipples, or genitals.

1. **Standing or Bent Over**:

- Standing positions, such as leaning against a wall or furniture, or bending over a surface, offer novelty and excitement. These positions allow for deeper penetration, different angles, and a sense of spontaneity.
- Variations: Experiment with height differences, angles, and support for comfort and stability. Use handholds or furniture for leverage and balance.

1. **Chair or Sitting Positions**:

- Sitting positions, such as straddling the penetrating partner in a chair or on a flat surface, offer intimate contact, eye contact, and control over depth and pace of penetration.
- Variations: Explore different seating positions, angles, and movements for added stimulation and pleasure. Incorporate kissing, touching, and communication to enhance intimacy.

Techniques for Enhanced Pleasure

1. **Clitoral and Penile Stimulation**:

- Incorporate manual or oral stimulation of the clitoris or penis during penetrative sex to enhance arousal, pleasure, and orgasmic potential for both partners.
- Use fingers, tongues, or sex toys designed for clitoral or penile stimulation to add variety and intensity to sexual experiences.

1. **G-Spot and Prostate Stimulation**:

- Experiment with positions and techniques that target the G-spot (located inside the vagina on the front wall) or prostate (located inside the rectum).
- Positions such as missionary with a pillow under the receiving partner's hips, cowgirl/reverse cowgirl with a curved motion, or doggy style with a G-spot or prostate toy can enhance stimulation and pleasure.

1. **Rhythm and Pace**:

- Vary the rhythm, pace, and intensity of thrusting or movements to build anticipation, prolong arousal, and enhance pleasure.
- Incorporate slow, teasing movements followed by faster, rhythmic thrusts to create a dynamic and pleasurable experience.

1. **Breath and Communication**:

- Focus on synchronized breathing, moans, and vocalizations to enhance arousal, connection, and communication during sexual encounters.
- Communicate openly about likes, dislikes, preferences, and adjustments to ensure mutual pleasure and comfort.

1. **Erotic Touch and Sensory Play**:

- Explore erotic touch, sensory play, and erogenous zones beyond genital stimulation. Incorporate kissing, nibbling, biting, massage, or sensory toys for heightened arousal and pleasure.
- Pay attention to feedback, cues, and reactions from your partner to tailor sensations and experiences for mutual enjoyment.

Tips for Safe and Comfortable Sex

1. **Use Lubrication**:

- Incorporate water-based or silicone-based lubricants to enhance comfort, reduce friction, and prevent discomfort or pain during sexual activity.
- Communicate with your partner about preferences for lubrication and adjust as needed for smooth and pleasurable experiences.

1. **Practice Safe Sex**:

- Use condoms or other barrier methods to prevent sexually transmitted infections (STIs) and unintended pregnancy. Condoms also reduce sensitivity, allowing for longer-lasting sexual activity.
- Communicate about STI testing, contraception options, and sexual health practices with your partner for a safe and responsible sexual experience.

1. **Listen to Your Body**:

- Pay attention to physical sensations, comfort levels, and any signs of discomfort or pain during sexual activity. Communicate openly with your partner and make adjustments as needed for a comfortable and enjoyable experience.

- Respect your own boundaries and communicate them to your partner. Consent and mutual respect are fundamental in sexual exploration and enjoyment.

Conclusion

Exploring sexual positions and techniques offers a pathway to enhanced pleasure, intimacy, and satisfaction in sexual encounters. By understanding different positions, incorporating varied techniques, and prioritizing communication and mutual pleasure, individuals and couples can create fulfilling and enjoyable sexual experiences. Experimentation, openness, and creativity in the bedroom contribute to a dynamic and satisfying sex life. It's important to prioritize comfort, safety, and consent during sexual exploration and to communicate openly with your partner about desires, boundaries, and preferences for a positive and mutually satisfying experience.

Twelve

Chapter 12: Performance Anxiety and Confidence

Performance anxiety and confidence are common factors that can impact male sexual health and well-being. This chapter explores the causes, effects, and strategies for managing performance anxiety, enhancing sexual confidence, and promoting a positive mindset for fulfilling sexual experiences.

Understanding Performance Anxiety

1. **Definition of Performance Anxiety**:

- Performance anxiety refers to feelings of stress, pressure, or self-doubt related to sexual performance, including concerns about achieving or maintaining an erection, satisfying a partner, or performing well sexually.
- It can manifest as physical symptoms (such as rapid heartbeat, sweating, or tension), psychological distress, and negative thoughts or beliefs about one's sexual abilities.

1. **Causes of Performance Anxiety**:

- Psychological Factors: Anxiety, stress, fear of failure, perfectionism, negative self-talk, past sexual experiences, or performance expectations can contribute to performance anxiety.
- Relationship Dynamics: Relationship conflicts, communication issues, lack of trust, or emotional disconnection with a partner can exacerbate performance anxiety.
- Physical Health: Health conditions (such as erectile dysfunction, premature ejaculation, or medical issues affecting sexual function), medication side effects, substance use, or fatigue can also influence performance anxiety.

Effects of Performance Anxiety

1. **Impact on Sexual Function**:

- Performance anxiety can interfere with sexual arousal, erection quality, ejaculatory control, and overall sexual function. It may lead to difficulties in achieving or maintaining an erection (erectile dysfunction), premature ejaculation, or inhibited sexual desire.
- Negative self-perception and fear of sexual inadequacy can further exacerbate anxiety and affect sexual confidence.

1. **Emotional and Psychological Consequences**:

- Performance anxiety can contribute to feelings of frustration, embarrassment, shame, guilt, or low self-esteem. It may lead to avoidance of sexual intimacy, relationship strain, or decreased sexual satisfaction for both partners.
- Persistent performance anxiety can impact mental well-being, self-image, and overall quality of life, highlighting the importance of addressing and managing anxiety effectively.

Strategies for Managing Performance Anxiety

1. **Communication and Education**:

- Openly discuss concerns, fears, and anxieties about sexual performance with your partner in a supportive and understanding manner. Communication fosters trust, reduces pressure, and promotes a collaborative approach to addressing anxiety.
- Educate yourself and your partner about sexual health, common sexual concerns, and realistic expectations. Understanding that occasional challenges are normal can alleviate anxiety and promote a positive mindset.

1. **Mindfulness and Relaxation Techniques**:

- Practice mindfulness techniques, such as deep breathing, meditation, progressive muscle relaxation, or guided imagery, to reduce stress, anxiety, and physical tension during sexual encounters.
- Incorporate relaxation exercises into daily routines to cultivate a sense of calm, presence, and self-awareness, which can enhance confidence and reduce performance-related worries.

1. **Cognitive Behavioral Therapy (CBT)**:

- Consider cognitive behavioral therapy (CBT) or counseling to address underlying beliefs, thought patterns, and behavioral responses related to performance anxiety.
- CBT techniques, such as cognitive restructuring, challenging negative thoughts, and exposure therapy, can help reframe perspectives, build confidence, and develop coping strategies for managing anxiety.

1. **Gradual Exposure and Sensate Focus**:

- Gradually expose yourself to sexual stimuli, sensations, or activities in a controlled and supportive environment to desensitize anxiety triggers and build confidence.
- Sensate focus exercises, involving non-genital touch and exploration with a partner, can promote relaxation, intimacy, and sensory awareness, reducing performance pressure.

1. **Healthy Lifestyle Habits**:

- Prioritize overall health and well-being through regular exercise, balanced nutrition, adequate sleep, and stress management practices. Physical well-being contributes to mental resilience, energy levels, and confidence.
- Limit alcohol consumption, avoid recreational drugs, and manage medication use responsibly, as substance abuse or misuse can exacerbate anxiety and affect sexual function.

Enhancing Sexual Confidence

1. **Positive Self-Talk and Beliefs**:

- Challenge negative self-talk and beliefs about sexual performance by focusing on strengths, past successes, and realistic expectations. Replace self-criticism with affirmations, encouragement, and self-compassion.
- Acknowledge that sexual experiences are varied, and occasional challenges do not define your overall sexual abilities or worth.

1. **Self-Exploration and Sexual Empowerment**:

- Explore your own body, pleasure zones, and erogenous areas through solo exploration, self-touch, or self-pleasure techniques. Understanding your own arousal patterns and preferences can boost sexual confidence.
- Experiment with different masturbation techniques, fantasies, or erotic

materials to enhance self-awareness, pleasure, and comfort with sexual experiences.

1. **Sensual and Non-Sexual Intimacy**:

- Prioritize non-sexual forms of intimacy, such as cuddling, kissing, affectionate touch, or shared activities, to deepen emotional connection and intimacy with your partner.
- Emphasize sensual experiences and mutual pleasure beyond performance-based goals, fostering a sense of connection, relaxation, and enjoyment in sexual encounters.

1. **Sexual Education and Skill Building**:

- Seek sexual education resources, books, workshops, or online courses focused on enhancing sexual skills, communication, and pleasure. Knowledge and skills development can boost confidence and competence in sexual interactions.
- Practice sexual techniques, communication skills, and mutual exploration with a partner in a supportive and non-judgmental environment, emphasizing pleasure, connection, and mutual satisfaction.

Overcoming Performance Pressure

1. **Focus on Sensations and Connection**:

- Shift the focus from performance goals or outcomes to present-moment sensations, connection with your partner, and shared pleasure. Emphasize intimacy, enjoyment, and mutual satisfaction rather than performance benchmarks.
- Practice mindfulness during sexual encounters, staying present, and attuned to sensations, emotions, and partner cues, which can reduce anxiety and enhance pleasure.

1. **Embrace Imperfections and Vulnerability**:

- Accept that imperfections, occasional challenges, and vulnerability are natural parts of sexual experiences. Embrace vulnerability as an opportunity for growth, learning, and deeper connection with your partner.
- Communicate openly about vulnerabilities, fears, and insecurities with your partner, fostering empathy, understanding, and mutual support in addressing performance anxiety.

1. **Seek Professional Support**:

- If performance anxiety persists despite self-help strategies, consider consulting a healthcare provider, therapist, or sex counselor experienced in addressing sexual concerns.
- Professional support can offer personalized guidance, therapeutic interventions, and strategies for managing anxiety, building confidence, and enhancing sexual well-being.

Conclusion

Performance anxiety and confidence play significant roles in male sexual health and satisfaction. By understanding the causes and effects of performance anxiety, implementing strategies for managing anxiety, enhancing sexual confidence, and fostering a positive mindset, individuals can navigate challenges and enjoy fulfilling sexual experiences. Open communication, education, mindfulness, self-exploration, and professional support are valuable tools in addressing performance anxiety and promoting sexual confidence. Remember that sexual experiences are diverse, and prioritizing mutual pleasure, connection, and well-being contributes to a healthy and satisfying sex life.

Thirteen

Chapter 13: Sexual Health Screenings and Check-ups

This chapter focuses on the importance of regular sexual health screenings and check-ups for males. It covers various aspects of sexual health examinations, testing procedures, preventive measures, and the role of healthcare providers in promoting sexual well-being.

Importance of Sexual Health Screenings

1. **Early Detection of STIs:**

- Regular sexual health screenings help detect sexually transmitted infections (STIs) early, allowing for prompt treatment and management. Many STIs may not present symptoms initially, making screenings crucial for early detection and prevention of complications.
- Common STIs include chlamydia, gonorrhea, syphilis, HIV/AIDS, herpes, human papillomavirus (HPV), and hepatitis B and C.

1. **Preventive Care:**

- Sexual health screenings are part of preventive care measures aimed at maintaining overall health and well-being. They enable healthcare providers to assess risk factors, provide education on safe sex practices, and offer guidance on sexual health maintenance.
- Regular screenings contribute to informed decision-making, risk reduction, and proactive management of sexual health concerns.

1. **Promotion of Sexual Well-Being**:

- Sexual health screenings promote sexual well-being by addressing concerns related to sexual function, reproductive health, contraception, fertility, and intimacy. They facilitate discussions on sexual health goals, preferences, and individualized care plans.
- Healthcare providers play a crucial role in promoting sexual health awareness, empowerment, and access to comprehensive sexual healthcare services.

Components of Sexual Health Screenings

1. **Medical History and Risk Assessment**:

- Healthcare providers conduct a comprehensive medical history review, including sexual history, contraceptive use, past STI diagnoses or treatments, vaccination status (e.g., HPV, hepatitis), and sexual health concerns.
- Risk assessment involves evaluating factors such as sexual activity, number of sexual partners, condom use, substance use, history of STIs, and potential exposure to STI risk factors.

1. **Physical Examination**:

- A physical examination may include genital inspection, examination of the anus and rectum (for individuals at risk of anal STIs), assessment of

lymph nodes, and evaluation of any visible signs or symptoms of STIs.
- Healthcare providers may also perform a pelvic examination for individuals assigned female at birth (AFAB) to assess reproductive health, including cervical cancer screening (Pap smear) and pelvic organ health.

1. **Laboratory Testing**:

- Laboratory testing is a key component of sexual health screenings and may include blood tests, urine tests, and swabs of genital, anal, or oral sites to detect STIs or assess sexual health markers.
- Common tests include screening for HIV, syphilis, gonorrhea, chlamydia, herpes simplex virus (HSV), HPV (for cervical cancer screening), hepatitis B and C, and other relevant STIs based on risk factors and symptoms.

1. **Counseling and Education**:

- Sexual health screenings provide an opportunity for counseling, education, and risk reduction strategies. Healthcare providers offer guidance on safer sex practices, condom use, STI prevention, contraception options, vaccination recommendations (e.g., HPV, hepatitis), and pre-exposure prophylaxis (PrEP) for HIV prevention.
- Counseling also addresses sexual health concerns, relationship dynamics, mental health aspects, fertility considerations, and sexual function issues, promoting holistic sexual well-being.

Recommended Frequency of Screenings

1. **General Guidelines**:

- The frequency of sexual health screenings depends on individual risk factors, sexual activity levels, age, sexual orientation, and healthcare provider recommendations.
- For sexually active individuals, routine annual screenings or screenings

at least once a year are generally recommended, even in the absence of symptoms or known exposure to STIs.

1. **High-Risk Populations**:

- High-risk populations, such as individuals with multiple sexual partners, history of STIs, inconsistent condom use, substance use, or engaging in high-risk sexual behaviors (e.g., unprotected anal sex), may require more frequent screenings or targeted testing based on risk assessment.

1. **Age-Specific Recommendations**:

- Adolescents and young adults should receive comprehensive sexual health education, screenings, and vaccinations as part of routine preventive care.
- Individuals aged 25 and older may undergo cervical cancer screening (Pap smear) as part of sexual health examinations, with screening intervals determined by guidelines and individual risk factors.

Common Sexual Health Tests and Examinations

1. **STI Testing**:

- STI testing typically includes screenings for chlamydia, gonorrhea, syphilis, HIV, herpes (HSV), hepatitis B and C, and HPV (for cervical cancer screening). Testing methods may involve blood tests, urine tests, swabs of genital or anal sites, and molecular tests (e.g., nucleic acid amplification tests).
- Testing may also include partner notification and treatment to prevent reinfection and transmission.

1. **HIV Testing**:

- HIV testing is essential for early detection, treatment initiation, and

prevention of HIV/AIDS transmission. Testing may involve blood tests, rapid HIV tests (oral or finger prick), or home self-testing kits.
- Regular HIV testing is recommended for sexually active individuals, individuals with multiple partners, injection drug users, men who have sex with men (MSM), and individuals at increased risk of HIV exposure.

1. **Cervical Cancer Screening**:

- Cervical cancer screening (Pap smear) is recommended for individuals with a cervix (AFAB) to detect abnormal cervical cell changes that may indicate precancerous or cancerous conditions.
- Screening intervals and methods may vary based on age, risk factors, vaccination status (HPV vaccine), and previous screening results.

1. **Genital Examination**:

- Genital examinations involve visual inspection, palpation, and assessment of the genital area, including the penis, scrotum, testicles, vulva, vagina, and perianal region. Healthcare providers check for signs of STIs, genital warts, lesions, or abnormalities.
- Anal and rectal examinations may be performed for individuals at risk of anal STIs or anal cancer, such as MSM or individuals with a history of anal intercourse.

Special Considerations and Preventive Measures

1. **Vaccinations**:

- Vaccinations play a crucial role in preventing certain STIs and related health conditions. Recommended vaccines include the HPV vaccine (for cervical cancer prevention and genital warts), hepatitis B vaccine, and hepatitis A vaccine for at-risk populations.
- Healthcare providers may recommend vaccination against HPV for

individuals aged 9-26, hepatitis B vaccination for adolescents and adults, and catch-up vaccinations based on individual risk factors.

1. **Pre-Exposure Prophylaxis (PrEP)**:

- PrEP involves taking antiretroviral medication (e.g., tenofovir/emtric-itabine) daily to reduce the risk of HIV infection in individuals at high risk of HIV exposure, such as MSM, individuals with HIV-positive partners, or individuals engaging in high-risk sexual behaviors.
- PrEP use requires regular follow-up visits, HIV testing, kidney function monitoring, and adherence to medication regimens under healthcare provider supervision.

1. **Safer Sex Practices**:

- Encourage and educate individuals on safer sex practices, including consistent and correct condom use, mutual monogamy, regular STI screenings, communication about sexual health with partners, and avoiding high-risk behaviors (e.g., unprotected sex, sharing needles).
- Discuss strategies for risk reduction, negotiation of condom use, and addressing barriers to safer sex practices in a non-judgmental and supportive manner.

Role of Healthcare Providers

1. **Comprehensive Sexual Health Assessment**:

- Healthcare providers conduct comprehensive sexual health assessments, screenings, and examinations tailored to individual needs, preferences, and risk factors.
- They offer non-judgmental, confidential, and culturally sensitive care, addressing sexual health concerns, providing education, and empowering individuals to make informed decisions about their sexual well-being.

1. **Education and Counseling**:

- Healthcare providers offer education, counseling, and resources on sexual health topics, including STI prevention, contraception options, reproductive health, sexual function, fertility considerations, and sexual satisfaction.
- They promote open communication, informed consent, autonomy, and empowerment in sexual health decision-making, fostering a collaborative patient-provider relationship.

1. **Treatment and Follow-up Care**:

- In cases of positive STI results or sexual health concerns, healthcare providers offer appropriate treatment, referrals, and follow-up care. They ensure confidentiality, respect privacy, and provide support throughout the care process.
- Follow-up visits, retesting, treatment adherence, and risk reduction counseling are part of ongoing sexual health management and preventive care.

Conclusion

Regular sexual health screenings and check-ups are essential components of preventive care, promoting early detection, treatment, and management of STIs, reproductive health concerns, and sexual well-being. By engaging in comprehensive sexual health assessments, discussing risk factors, implementing preventive measures, and fostering open communication with healthcare providers, individuals can prioritize their sexual health and make informed decisions about their sexual well-being. Healthcare providers play a crucial role in offering non-judgmental, culturally competent, and patient-centered sexual healthcare services, empowering individuals to take charge of their sexual health and lead fulfilling, healthy lives.

Fourteen

Chapter 14: Age and Sexual Health

This chapter explores the relationship between age and sexual health, highlighting the impact of aging on sexual function, intimacy, reproductive health, and overall well-being. It addresses common age-related changes, challenges, and strategies for maintaining sexual health and satisfaction throughout different life stages.

Age-Related Changes in Sexual Health

1. **Hormonal Changes**:

- Hormonal fluctuations, particularly in testosterone levels for males, can affect libido, erectile function, and sexual desire. Age-related declines in testosterone production may contribute to changes in sexual arousal and performance.
- Females may experience hormonal changes related to menopause, leading to decreased estrogen levels, vaginal dryness, changes in libido, and potential discomfort during intercourse.

1. **Physical Changes**:

- Aging can result in physical changes that impact sexual health, such as changes in muscle tone, flexibility, joint mobility, and cardiovascular health. These factors can influence sexual stamina, comfort during sexual activities, and overall physical fitness for sexual function.
- Chronic health conditions, medication side effects, and age-related ailments (such as arthritis, diabetes, or cardiovascular disease) may also affect sexual function and satisfaction.

1. **Psychological and Emotional Factors**:

- Psychological and emotional factors play a significant role in sexual health across different age groups. Aging may bring about changes in body image, self-esteem, stress levels, mental health, and relationship dynamics, which can influence sexual desire, intimacy, and satisfaction.
- Addressing emotional well-being, communication, and relationship dynamics is crucial for promoting sexual health and satisfaction as individuals age.

Age-Specific Considerations

1. **Young Adults (18-35)**:

- Young adults may focus on exploring sexuality, forming intimate relationships, and establishing sexual identities. They may encounter challenges related to sexual experimentation, communication, contraception use, and STI prevention.
- Education on safe sex practices, contraception options, consent, communication skills, and healthy relationships is vital for promoting sexual health and well-being in young adults.

1. **Middle-Aged Adults (36-65)**:

- Middle-aged adults may face age-related changes in sexual function, such as changes in libido, erectile function, vaginal dryness, or menopausal symptoms. They may also navigate challenges related to work-life balance, stress, and relationship dynamics.

- Encouraging regular sexual health screenings, addressing age-related health concerns (e.g., cardiovascular health, diabetes management), and promoting intimacy and communication with partners are important for sexual health in this age group.

1. **Older Adults (65+):**

- Older adults may experience age-related changes in sexual function, physical mobility, and chronic health conditions that impact sexual health. They may also encounter social stigma, myths, and misconceptions about aging and sexuality.
- Emphasizing sexual health as an integral part of overall well-being, addressing age-related health concerns (e.g., bone health, cognitive function), promoting sexual pleasure and intimacy, and providing access to age-friendly sexual healthcare services are essential for older adults' sexual well-being.

Strategies for Maintaining Sexual Health Across Ages

1. **Regular Sexual Health Screenings:**

- Engage in regular sexual health screenings and check-ups to assess sexual function, STI risk, hormonal balance, and overall reproductive health. Consult healthcare providers for age-appropriate screenings, vaccinations, and preventive care.

1. **Healthy Lifestyle Habits:**

- Adopt a healthy lifestyle that includes regular exercise, balanced nutrition, adequate sleep, stress management, and moderation in alcohol consumption and tobacco use. Physical fitness and overall well-being contribute to sexual function and vitality.

- Manage chronic health conditions effectively, follow medication regimens as prescribed, and communicate with healthcare providers about any concerns or side effects impacting sexual health.

1. **Communication and Intimacy**:

- Prioritize open communication, emotional intimacy, and connection with partners. Discuss sexual desires, preferences, concerns, and changes in sexual function openly and without judgment.
- Explore new ways to enhance intimacy, such as non-sexual affection, communication skills, sensual touch, shared activities, and mutual exploration of sexual desires.

1. **Sexual Education and Resources**:

- Stay informed about sexual health topics, age-related changes in sexual function, contraception options, STI prevention, and sexual pleasure techniques. Seek reputable sexual education resources, workshops, or counseling as needed.
- Access age-friendly sexual healthcare services that offer tailored assessments, education, counseling, and support for age-related sexual health concerns.

1. **Adaptation and Flexibility**:

- Be adaptable and flexible in sexual activities, exploring new techniques, positions, and adjustments to accommodate age-related changes or physical limitations. Focus on pleasure, connection, and mutual satisfaction rather than performance-oriented goals.
- Experiment with sensual touch, erotic communication, fantasy exploration, and intimacy-building activities that promote sexual well-being

and fulfillment across different life stages.

Addressing Age-Related Sexual Concerns

1. **Erectile Dysfunction (ED)**:

- Erectile dysfunction is a common age-related concern for males, characterized by difficulty achieving or maintaining an erection sufficient for sexual activity. It can be caused by physical factors (e.g., cardiovascular disease, diabetes, hormonal imbalances), psychological factors (e.g., stress, anxiety, depression), or a combination of both.
- Consult healthcare providers for assessment, diagnosis, and management of erectile dysfunction. Treatment options may include lifestyle changes, medication (e.g., phosphodiesterase inhibitors), vacuum erection devices, penile implants, or counseling.

1. **Menopause and Hormonal Changes**:

- Menopause, typically occurring in females aged 45-55, involves hormonal changes, such as decreased estrogen levels, leading to symptoms like hot flashes, vaginal dryness, mood changes, and changes in sexual desire. These changes can impact sexual function and comfort during intercourse.
- Discuss menopausal symptoms and sexual health concerns with healthcare providers. Hormone replacement therapy (HRT), vaginal moisturizers, lubricants, and counseling may be recommended to alleviate symptoms and enhance sexual comfort.

1. **Chronic Health Conditions**:

- Chronic health conditions, such as cardiovascular disease, diabetes, obesity, hypertension, and arthritis, can affect sexual health and function. These conditions may impact blood flow, nerve function, hormonal balance, or physical mobility, influencing sexual desire, arousal, and performance.

- Manage chronic health conditions effectively through medication adherence, lifestyle modifications (e.g., healthy diet, regular exercise, weight management), stress reduction, and regular healthcare monitoring. Communicate with healthcare providers about any sexual concerns related to chronic conditions for personalized care.

1. **Sexual Desire and Intimacy**:

- Changes in sexual desire and intimacy are common with aging and may vary based on individual preferences, relationship dynamics, and life circumstances. It's normal for sexual desire to fluctuate over time, and maintaining emotional intimacy and connection is key to sexual satisfaction.
- Prioritize emotional connection, communication, and mutual understanding with partners. Explore ways to enhance intimacy through shared activities, quality time together, affectionate touch, and open conversations about sexual desires and needs.

Promoting Sexual Wellness Across the Lifespan

1. **Education and Awareness**:

- Promote sexual health education, awareness, and destigmatization of age-related sexual concerns. Encourage open conversations about sexuality, aging, and sexual well-being in families, communities, and healthcare settings.
- Provide age-appropriate sexual education resources, workshops, and support groups for individuals of all ages to address sexual health needs and promote positive attitudes toward sexuality throughout life.

1. **Access to Sexual Healthcare Services**:

- Advocate for accessible, inclusive, and age-friendly sexual healthcare services that address diverse sexual health needs across different age groups. Ensure healthcare providers receive training on age-related sexual health concerns, communication skills, and cultural competence.
- Empower individuals to seek sexual healthcare services, screenings, and consultations without fear of stigma, discrimination, or judgment, promoting proactive management of sexual health and well-being.

1. **Research and Innovation**:

- Support research initiatives, innovation, and advancements in age-related sexual health, including treatments for sexual dysfunction, age-friendly sexual healthcare models, technology-based interventions, and holistic approaches to sexual wellness.
- Encourage collaboration among healthcare professionals, researchers, policymakers, and community organizations to address gaps in sexual health care, promote best practices, and improve outcomes for individuals of all ages.

Conclusion

Age is a significant factor in sexual health, influencing sexual function, intimacy, reproductive health, and overall well-being across different life stages. By understanding age-related changes, challenges, and strategies for maintaining sexual health, individuals can prioritize their sexual well-being and lead fulfilling, satisfying lives. Open communication, education, regular sexual health screenings, healthy lifestyle habits, adaptation to changes, and access to age-friendly sexual healthcare services are essential components of promoting sexual wellness across the lifespan. Empowering individuals to embrace their sexuality, address age-related concerns, and seek support when needed contributes to a positive and holistic approach to sexual health and well-being.

Fifteen

Chapter 15: Resources and Support

This chapter provides a comprehensive overview of resources, support services, and tools available to individuals seeking information, guidance, and assistance related to sexual health. It covers a range of resources, including educational materials, online platforms, support groups, healthcare services, and advocacy organizations dedicated to promoting sexual well-being.

Educational Resources

1. **Books and Publications**:

- Numerous books and publications cover various aspects of sexual health, including reproductive health, STI prevention, sexual function, intimacy, LGBTQ+ issues, and sexual pleasure. Recommended titles include "The Guide to Getting It On" by Paul Joannides, "Come as You Are" by Emily Nagoski, and "The Ultimate Guide to Sex and Disability" by Miriam Kaufman, Cory Silverberg, and Fran Odette.
- These resources provide evidence-based information, practical tips, personal narratives, and empowerment strategies for individuals of all ages and backgrounds.

1. **Online Articles and Websites**:

- Online platforms such as Planned Parenthood, Mayo Clinic, WebMD, Healthline, and the American Sexual Health Association (ASHA) offer comprehensive articles, fact sheets, FAQs, and resources on sexual health topics. These resources cover sexual education, contraception options, STI information, sexual dysfunction, relationship advice, and sexual pleasure tips.
- Verified and reputable websites provide accurate, up-to-date information, guidance on seeking healthcare services, and tools for self-assessment and education.

1. **Sexual Health Courses and Workshops**:

- Online courses, workshops, and webinars on sexual health topics are available through platforms like Coursera, Udemy, and local community centers or healthcare organizations. These courses cover diverse topics such as sexual education, communication skills, STI prevention, contraception, sexual pleasure techniques, and intimacy-building strategies.
- Participating in sexual health courses promotes knowledge, skills development, and empowerment in managing sexual well-being and relationships.

Online Platforms and Apps

1. **Sexual Health Apps**:

- Mobile applications focused on sexual health offer features such as STI risk assessment, contraception reminders, menstrual cycle tracking, sexual education modules, sexual pleasure guides, and access to tele-health services. Examples include Planned Parenthood Direct, Clue, MySexDoctor, and BedSider.
- These apps provide convenient tools for self-assessment, education,

communication with healthcare providers, and monitoring sexual health parameters.

1. **Telehealth and Virtual Consultations**:

- Telehealth platforms connect individuals with healthcare providers for virtual consultations, confidential discussions about sexual health concerns, STI testing, contraception prescriptions, and sexual dysfunction assessments. Telehealth services offer convenience, accessibility, and privacy for seeking sexual healthcare.
- Telehealth providers include Planned Parenthood, Nurx, Lemonaid Health, and local healthcare systems offering telemedicine options.

1. **Online Support Communities**:

- Online forums, social media groups, and community platforms facilitate peer support, information sharing, and discussions on sexual health topics. Platforms like Reddit (subreddits such as r/sex, r/sexover30), HealthUnlocked, and online support groups organized by advocacy organizations offer spaces for individuals to ask questions, share experiences, and access resources.
- Engaging in online support communities fosters connection, reduces stigma, and provides a sense of belonging and understanding for individuals navigating sexual health challenges.

Healthcare Services

1. **Sexual Health Clinics**:

- Sexual health clinics, such as those affiliated with Planned Parenthood, community health centers, LGBTQ+ healthcare providers, and specialized sexual health clinics, offer comprehensive sexual healthcare services. These services include STI testing, contraception counseling,

reproductive health screenings, sexual dysfunction evaluations, LGBTQ+ affirming care, and sexual health education.
- Sexual health clinics prioritize confidentiality, non-judgmental care, culturally competent services, and access to affordable or sliding-scale payment options for individuals seeking sexual healthcare.

1. **STI Testing and Treatment Centers**:

- STI testing and treatment centers provide confidential testing, diagnosis, treatment, and counseling for sexually transmitted infections. Local health departments, community clinics, and private healthcare providers offer STI screenings for chlamydia, gonorrhea, syphilis, HIV, herpes, HPV, and hepatitis.
- Timely STI testing and treatment are crucial for early detection, prevention of complications, partner notification, and reducing STI transmission rates.

1. **Reproductive Health Services**:

- Reproductive health services encompass contraception options, family planning counseling, pregnancy testing, abortion care, fertility evaluations, preconception counseling, and reproductive healthcare screenings. Healthcare providers specializing in reproductive health offer personalized care plans based on individual needs, preferences, and reproductive goals.
- Access to reproductive health services promotes informed decision-making, contraceptive choices, pregnancy prevention, and support for reproductive health concerns.

Support Groups and Counseling Services

1. **Sexual Health Support Groups**:

- Support groups focused on sexual health provide a safe space for individuals to share experiences, receive peer support, access information, and discuss sexual health concerns. These groups may address topics such as STI stigma, sexual dysfunction, LGBTQ+ affirming care, sexual trauma recovery, and relationship challenges.
- Local community centers, advocacy organizations, mental health providers, and online platforms host sexual health support groups and counseling services tailored to diverse populations and needs.

1. **Sex Therapy and Counseling**:

- Sex therapists, counselors, and mental health professionals specializing in sexual health offer individual, couples, or group therapy sessions to address sexual concerns, intimacy issues, communication challenges, sexual trauma, and relationship dynamics.
- Sex therapy emphasizes education, communication skills, intimacy-building strategies, emotional connection, and holistic approaches to sexual well-being and satisfaction.

1. **Hotlines and Crisis Intervention**:

- Hotlines and crisis intervention services provide immediate support, information, counseling, and referrals for individuals experiencing sexual health crises, emergencies, or mental health concerns. Crisis hotlines may focus on topics such as sexual assault, domestic violence, LGBTQ+ support, suicide prevention, and mental health crises.
- Organizations such as RAINN (Rape, Abuse & Incest National Network), National Domestic Violence Hotline, The Trevor Project, and crisis intervention centers offer confidential, 24/7 support services for individuals

in need.

Advocacy Organizations and Resources

1. **Sexual Health Advocacy Organizations**:

- Advocacy organizations dedicated to sexual health promote education, awareness, advocacy, and policy initiatives addressing sexual health rights, access to healthcare, stigma reduction, and comprehensive sexual education. Examples include Planned Parenthood, The American Sexual Health Association (ASHA), Advocates for Youth, and the Guttmacher Institute.
- These organizations offer resources, advocacy tools, policy research, grassroots campaigns, and community outreach efforts to advance sexual health equity, inclusivity, and empowerment.

1. **LGBTQ+ Health Resources**:

- LGBTQ+ health organizations and resources provide specialized support, affirming care, education, and advocacy for LGBTQ+ individuals' sexual health needs. Organizations such as GLAAD, The Trevor Project, National LGBTQ+ Health Education Center, and local LGBTQ+ community centers offer resources on sexual health, identity affirmation, cultural competence, and healthcare access.
- LGBTQ+ affirming healthcare providers, support groups, and resources promote inclusive sexual health services, non-discrimination policies, and culturally competent care for LGBTQ+ communities.

1. **Sexual Health Campaigns and Initiatives**:

- Sexual health campaigns, initiatives, and awareness-raising efforts promote public education, destigmatization of sexual health topics, consent culture, healthy relationships, and access to sexual healthcare services.

Campaigns may focus on STI prevention, contraception awareness, reproductive rights, sexual violence prevention, and diversity in sexual health representation.

- Participating in sexual health campaigns, advocacy efforts, and community initiatives empowers individuals to contribute to positive change, challenge stigma, and promote sexual health equity and rights.

Conclusion

Resources and support for sexual health encompass a wide range of educational materials, online platforms, healthcare services, support groups, counseling options, advocacy organizations, and awareness campaigns dedicated to promoting sexual well-being and empowerment. By accessing reliable resources, seeking support from qualified professionals, engaging in education and advocacy efforts, and advocating for inclusive, equitable sexual healthcare services, individuals can prioritize their sexual health, make informed decisions, and navigate sexual health challenges with confidence and empowerment. Empowering individuals, promoting sexual health literacy, and fostering supportive communities contribute to a positive and holistic approach to sexual wellness and fulfillment.

Sixteen

Glossary

A - Abstinence: Refraining from sexual activity, often practiced for personal, religious, or health reasons.

B - Birth Control: Methods or devices used to prevent pregnancy, including condoms, hormonal contraception, and intrauterine devices (IUDs).

C - Consent: Voluntary, enthusiastic agreement to engage in sexual activity, based on clear communication and mutual understanding.

D - Desire: A person's emotional or physical longing for sexual intimacy or arousal.

E - Empowerment: The process of gaining knowledge, confidence, and autonomy to make informed decisions about one's sexual health and well-being.

F - Fertility: The ability to conceive and reproduce, influenced by factors such as age, hormonal balance, and reproductive health.

G - Gender Identity: A person's internal sense of their gender, which may differ from their assigned sex at birth.

H - Healthy Relationships: Relationships characterized by mutual respect, communication, trust, and consent, contributing to emotional and sexual well-being.

I - Intimacy: Emotional, physical, or sexual closeness and connection between individuals, fostering emotional bonds and trust.

J - Judgment-Free: Providing information, support, and services without stigma, shame, or judgment based on sexual preferences or behaviors.

K - Knowledge: Understanding of sexual anatomy, physiology, reproductive health, contraception options, STI prevention, and sexual pleasure.

L - LGBTQ+: Acronym for lesbian, gay, bisexual, transgender, queer/questioning, and other identities, acknowledging diverse sexual orientations and gender identities.

M - Menopause: Natural cessation of menstruation and reproductive capacity in individuals assigned female at birth, typically occurring in midlife.

N - Non-Monogamy: Relationship style involving consensual romantic or sexual connections with multiple partners, with transparency and communication.

O - Orgasm: Peak of sexual arousal characterized by intense physical pleasure and release, often accompanied by muscle contractions.

P - Pleasure: Positive, enjoyable sensations experienced during sexual activities, contributing to overall sexual satisfaction and well-being.

Q - Queer: Umbrella term encompassing diverse sexual orientations and gender identities outside heteronormative norms, embracing fluidity and inclusivity.

R - Reproductive Health: Overall well-being of the reproductive system, encompassing fertility, contraception, pregnancy, childbirth, and reproductive rights.

S - STI/STD: Sexually transmitted infection/disease, infections transmitted through sexual contact, including HIV, chlamydia, gonorrhea, syphilis, herpes, and HPV.

T - Transgender: Individuals whose gender identity differs from their assigned sex at birth, often seeking gender-affirming medical care and social support.

U - Understanding: Awareness, knowledge, and empathy toward diverse sexual orientations, gender identities, sexual health needs, and experiences.

V - Values: Personal beliefs, principles, and attitudes that guide sexual decision-making, relationships, and behaviors.

W - Wellness: Holistic approach to health, encompassing physical, emotional, mental, and social aspects of well-being, including sexual health.

X - eXplore: Encouragement to explore and understand one's own sexuality, desires, boundaries, and preferences in a safe and consensual manner.

Y - Youth: Adolescents and young adults navigating sexual development, relationships, education, and reproductive health choices.

Z - Zero Judgment: Commitment to providing support, education, and resources without stigma, bias, or discrimination based on sexual orientation, gender identity, or sexual behaviors.

This glossary aims to provide clarity and understanding of key terms and concepts related to sexual health, promoting informed decision-making, communication, and empowerment for readers.